Bullying, Burnout, or Moral Injury?
The Many Faces of Democide
Your 28th Psychiatric Consultation
William R. Yee M.D., J.D.
Copyright Applied for 01/09/22

Table of Contents

Introduction: Democide

The reader will better understand the substance of this missive if the reader understands the context.

First, the reader should understand what Democide is.
Democide is the murder of citizens by the government. Democide is pervasive in government.

Governments kill their own citizens to assert power. Socrates is an example of selective democide.

Socrates, born 470 years before the birth of Christ in Athens, Greece and died 399 years before the birth of Christ in Athens Greece.

Socrates was an ancient Greek philosopher whose life and thought profoundly influences Western philosophy.

I suggest reading,
The Hemlock Cup: Socrates, Athens and the Search for the Good Life, February 14, 2012, by Bettany Hughes.

Socrates was murdered by his own government because he threatened the power of a few individuals in the government.
Socrates is an example of Old Wisdom, "No good deed goes unpunished."
Socrates is an example of the Butterfly Effect.

Each of us has the power by simply talking to create a huge and long-lasting effect on the future of the World. Your few words here and there can create another Butterfly Effect that changes the course of history.

For want of a nail the horse lacked a shoe.
For want of a shoe the soldier lacked a horse.
For want of a horse the cavalry lacked a man.
For want of a man the cavalry lost the battle.
For want of that battle the empire lost the war.
For want of a victory in the war the empire fell into ruins and was forgotten in the pages of history.

Rummel estimated that there have been 262 million victims of democide in the 20th century, From Wikipedia, the free encyclopedia

Genghis Khan is responsible for the Mongol Empire, and one estimate is that about 11% of the world's population was killed either during or immediately after the Mongol invasions (around 37.75–60 million people) https://en.wikipedia.org/wiki/Destruction_under_the_Mongol_Empire .

At some point conquerors become rulers and murder of citizens persists after war to sustain power and control.

Democide has many faces. Short of murder, taxation, imprisonment, exile to reservations, gun control, forced labor, organ harvesting, regulation of farming and businesses can add up to death by a thousand cuts, with no single cut sufficient to cause death.

Self-Organizing Systems

Another way of looking at government is through the lens of self-organizing systems.

Self-organizing systems are elements that interact according to a few simple rules in a manner that presents with the appearance of order and organization.

Self-organization occurs in many physical, chemical, biological, robotic, and cognitive systems.

Examples of self-organization include crystallization, thermal convection of fluids, chemical oscillation, animal swarming, neural circuits, and black markets.
From Wikipedia, the free encyclopedia.

Politics, the stock market, and most social organizations fall into the category of self-organizing systems.

The order is an illusion and allows for short term predictability that evaporates in attempts at long term predictability.

Attempts to maintain order are eventually defeated in strange and unpredictable ways.

An example is the fall of any empire or the fall of the Berlin Wall.

I suggest as an introduction to this topic: Emergence: The Connected Lives of Ants, Brains, Cities, and Software by Steven Johnson
Paperback – September 10, 2002

Politics, the weather, the stock market, businesses, governments, and medical facilities are examples of self-organizing systems. Chaos theory describes the mathematics of these systems.

Chaos Theory

 Chaos theory rests in nonlinear equations.
A linear equation has one unknown, any number of constants, and is limited to a power of one,

e.g., $X = bY + a$ where b and a are constants and the only unknown is the Y

A nonlinear equation has more than one unknown, and a power of 2 or more with any number of constants.

e.g., $X = aY^2 + bZ + c$

Where Y is an unknown to the power of 2 and Z is an unknown and a, b, and c are constants.

There are better explanations, and my explanation may be incorrect, although the substance is similar and sufficient to identify major differences between linear and nonlinear equations.

I suggest that the reader look at
Chaos: Making a New Science
Paperback – August 26, 2008
by James Gleick
Available on Amazon:
Audiobook 1 Credit Paperback $16.71
Available at Thriftbooks.com for 4.19

Nonlinear equations define Chaos Theory.

At a starting point there is stability.

However, nonlinear equations describe instability created by small differences or changes over time.

There are tipping points where a slight change can create a huge change. This is where the Butterfly Effect makes an impact.

Each individual in an organization has the power to create that slight change.

That small change is unpredictable in the long term.

The result is that the stock market, the weather, politics, suicide, and homicide are predictable in the short term, but unpredictable in the long term. Organizations cannot control the butterfly effect.

Organizations are unstable because all it takes is a divorce, a domestic quarrel, a stroke, a new baby, or a promotion, to change a member of the organization.

Any change can launch the Butterfly Effect. Control is an imaginary construct and an illusion in the fog of wishful thinking.

For an introduction I suggest,
Chaos and society A. Albert (Ed.). (1995). Chaos and society (Vol. 29). Ios Press. The literature is large, and the reader will be overwhelmed by the amount of literature available.

Suffice it to say. All healthcare facilities are very different, even though they all rely upon the same medications, the same surgeries, the same counseling techniques, the same DSM-V etc. Slight differences in personnel create a large difference in outcomes.
The rest of this book will describe small differences in starting points that result in large differences in outcomes.

Now for the rest of the story a' la Paul Harvey.

Bullying?

I am small, Chinese, and different.

I have been bullied all my life.

I never complained about it because I saw that it was pervasive and complaining seemed to do nothing but make it worse.

I do know bullying when I see it, and it is thinly veiled throughout the health care systems and society.

Minorities participate in the bullying, to th point that society is so fractured that there is no majority, and everybody is being bullied.

Most people have been bullied.
"About 6 of every 10 men (or 60%) and 5 of every 10 women (or 50%) experience at least one trauma in their lives"

PTSD: National Center for PTSD
https://www.ptsd.va.gov/understand/comm
on/cmmon_adults.asp

Nationwide, 81% of women and 43% of
men reported experiencing some form of
sexual harassment and/or assault in their
lifetime

National Sexual Violence Resource Center
(NSVRC) https://www.nsvrc.org/statistics

"National studies of U.S. adult men and
women, which found prevalence of direct
physical or sexual assault victimization to
be 55% among women and 66.8% among
men (Tjaden & Thoennes, 1998)."

National Estimates of Exposure to
Traumatic Events and PTSD Prevalence
Using DSM-IV and DSM-5 Criteria
Dean G. Kilpatrick, Heidi S. Resnick,
Melissa E. Milanak, Mark W. Miller,
Katherine M.
Keyes, and Matthew J. Friedman
J Trauma Stress. Author manuscript;
available in PMC 2014 Oct 1.

Published in final edited form as: J Trauma Stress. 2013 Oct; 26(5): 537–547.
doi: 10.1002/jts.21848
PMCID: PMC4096796
NIHMSID: NIHMS 596966 PMID: 24151000
https://www.ncbi.nlm.nih.gov/pmc/articles/PM4096796/

Bullies and Their Victims: Understanding a Pervasive Problem in the Schools
George M. Batsche &Howard M. Knoff
Pages 165-174 | Published online: 22 Dec 2019
https://doi.org/10.1080/02796015.1994.1208574

Bullying is Pervasive in
the Healthcare Setting.

"Poor staffing levels, excessive workloads, subpar management skills, stress and lack of autonomy are some of the factors that contribute to bullying in the workplace - including in medicine - according to a recent AMA report on the problem that pervades health care and how to stop it."

Why bullying happens in health care and how to stop it
Brendan Murphy
Senior News Writer
PHYSICIAN HEALTH
APR 2, 2021

Patients bully healthcare workers with threats, false accusations of neglect, abuse, and discrimination, and even assaults.

"Nearly 50% of emergency physicians say they've been assaulted. 70% of emergency nurses report being hit or kicked on the job. So, what's the solution?"
Rising violence in the emergency department
Ken Budd, Special to AAMC News
February 24, 2020

What is the solution to bullying?

The trends towards, understaffing, exploitation and abuse of healthcare workers have survived decades of putative "solutions."

Reducing workplace bullying in healthcare organizations
Randle, Jacqueline; Stevenson, Keith; Grayling, Ian; Walker, Christine.
Nursing Standard (through 2013); London
Vol. 21, Iss. 22, (Feb 7-Feb 13, 2007): 49-56; quiz 58

Every religion uses the Golden Rule, "do unto others as you would have them do unto you."

This is the cure to bullying.

Unfortunately, antisocial personalities and antisocial behaviors gain traction in social organizations.
With the unfair advantages of lying, stealing, cheating, intimidation, threats, and assaults the antisocial personalities have an unfair advantage in reaching the top.

"The lifetime prevalence of antisocial personality disorder (APD), conduct disorder, and adult antisocial behavior were 3.6%, 1.1%, and 12.3%, respectively.

Prevalence of alcohol use disorders and drug use disorders were
30.3% and 10.3%, respectively."

Prevalence, correlates, and comorbidity of DSM-IV antisocial personality syndromes and alcohol and specific drug use disorders in the United States: results from the national epidemiologic survey on alcohol and related conditions
Wilson M Compton 1, Kevin P Conway, Frederick S Stinson, James D Colliver, Bridget
F Grant
PMID: 15960559 DOI: 10.4088/jcp.v66n0602
The prevalence of addiction and intoxication in emergency rooms increases the risks of threats, abuse, and assaults directed at health care workers.

Burnout?

There has been a growing literature on professional burnout and the retirement of a large number of healthcare professionals which accelerated during the Covid-19 pandemic.

The issue of burnout and early retirement of healthcare professionals has been simmering for many years.

The loss of seasoned health care workers has resulted in the rise of EAP's, Employee Assistance Programs.

The employee receives evaluation, diagnosis, and treatment for a mental illness caused by the stress of working in an environment of a high patient case load, a heavy documentation burden, and short hours in which to accomplish the work.

An egregious example is nurses who were expected to work off the clock, after their eight-hour shift without pay to complete the paperwork,

Many nurses retired and then they were given higher pay and hired in greater numbers.

Creep, the tendency to add more patients with more paperwork, without additional time or pay tends to recreate the same problems over and over as MBAs, as administrators, attempt to control costs and increase profits.

This led to the EAP's (Employee Assistance Programs).

Hard work was rewarded with a diagnosis of a mental illness, medication, counseling, and an Employee Appreciation Day.

When it came time for re-licensure, application for malpractice insurance, review by the credentials committee for annual credentialling, the healthcare workers were burdened with responding to inquiries about mental illness and fitness for work as a healthcare professional.

No good deed goes unpunished?

Before Covid-19 there was literature on Burnout.

There were Employee Assistance programs. The health care worker was given an evaluation, a diagnosis of mental illness and treatment of mental illness. "46 percent of physicians," suffered burn out.

"Lower patient satisfaction and care quality,
Higher medical error rates and malpractice risk,
Higher physician and staff turnover,
Physician alcohol and drug abuse and addiction,
Physician suicide.

Yes, burnout can be a fatal disorder. Suicide rates for both men and women are higher in physicians than the general population and widely underreported.[9]"

Physician Burnout: Its Origin, Symptoms, and Five Main Causes Burnout is everywhere, but you can't fight an enemy unless you recognize it.
Dike Drummond, MD
Fam Pract Manag. 2015 Sep-Oct;22(5):42-47.

Covid-19 created a tipping point among healthcare workers.

"An overwhelming 55% of front-line health care workers reported burnout (defined as mental and physical exhaustion from chronic workplace stress)"
Medical burnout: Breaking bad
Dharam Kaushik, MD, June 4, 2021

Moral Injury?

Suddenly there was an epiphany.

Someone realized that most of the employees were stressed, but not mentally ill. The employees were struggling with bullying and a dysfunctional work environment.

Healthcare providers are expected to take care of the sick and dying.

However, the MBAs were administrators serving the stockholders first and the patients second and the employees third.

The administrative priorities were cost control, revenue stream, and profits.

As a result, the employees were struggling with many stakeholders in addition to the patient.

Clinicians, forced to consider the demands of other stakeholders - the electronic medical record (EMR), the insurers, the hospital, the health care system, the peer review committee, the malpractice insurance carrier, the state licensing board, the credentialling committee, the patient, the patient's family, the community, vocal self interest groups, the judge, the jury, the prosecutor, as other players force their way into the room with the clinician and the patient.

After the meeting, all the stakeholders complete a satisfaction survey.

The clinician has a peer review that includes the patient's response to treatment and the satisfaction of the patient and all the other stakeholder.

The joint commission, the hospital credentialling committee, the specialty medical boards, the electronic medical record, the risk management committee, and the peer review committee all add layers of documentation to be added during and after the visit.

Patient's, the putative primary beneficiaries, find that they spend time with clinicians who do not make eye contact, but have their faces buried into a computer screen during the "face to face," contact that is the basis for submitting billing to the insurance company?

Patient satisfaction goes down the toilet because of the documentation requirements.

Quality of care, well, the clinician is now a data entry clerk, and the administrative chain of command now can push a button and create impressive spreadsheets.

The administrators are looking real good.

The cash flow is really good.

Clients don't like their clinicians looking into the computers while talking to the clients.

'Death by 1000 Cuts': Medscape National Physician Burnout & Suicide Report 2021
Leslie Kane, MA | January 22, 2021
All material on this website is protected by copyright, Copyright © 1994-2022 by

Burnout is properly redefined as moral injury and "These routine, incessant betrayals of patient care and trust are examples of 'death by a thousand cuts.' Any one of them, delivered alone, might heal. But repeated on a daily basis, they coalesce into the moral injury of health care."

Physicians aren't 'burning out.' They're suffering from moral injury
By Simon G. Talbot and Wendy Dean
July 26, 2018
https://www.statnews.com/2018/07/26/phys icians-not-burning-out-they-are-suffering- moral-injury/

The healthcare system has been suffering from pressure to provide more paperwork and more care with fewer providers for decades.

Minimalist Management strategies taught in MBA programs is the primary driving force.

Minimalist Management is the practice of hiring the minimum number of people, who are the least qualified, and lowest paid to generate a revenue stream with minimal costs.

This results in health care services having a chain of command with non-physicians at the top because physicians are expensive.

Any time you put a non-physician supervisor between the CEO and the physician provider the revenue stream creates a disconnect between the best medical practice and the patient care.

"The number of physicians in the United States grew 150 percent between 1975 and 2010, roughly in keeping with population growth, while the number of healthcare administrators increased 3,200 percent for the same time period."

Expert Forum: The rise (and rise) of the healthcare administrator By Joe Cantlupe | November 7, 2017, https://www.athenahealth.com/knowledge-hub/ practice-management/expert-forum-rise-and-ris e-healthcare-administrator

The Great Healthcare Bloat: 10 Administrators for Every 1 U.S. Doctor https://www.healthline.com/health-news/policy- ten-administrators-for-every-one-us-doctor-092 813

"By far the biggest culprit of the mushrooming workload is the electronic medical record, or E.M.R. It has burrowed its tentacles into every aspect of the healthcare system."

The Business of Health Care Depends on Exploiting Doctors and Nurses
One resource seems infinite and free: the professionalism of caregivers.
June 8, 2019

Arbitrary time limits with the patient
does not allow for the best practice of
medicine.

The best practice requires a complete
assessment, even if the client is depressed,
confused, disorganized, speaks through
an interpreter and is slow to answer
questions.

The best practice requires informed
choice.

That means that time must be taken to
educate the client as to what the risks and
benefits are and time for the client to
make that choice.
Is the provider seeing 5, 10, 15, 20, 25, 30
"clients," a day?

At what point is the contact a fly by with
the work product a billable progress note,

a prescription and a mere salute to the best practice of informed choice?

Who in the chain of command sets the appointment schedule for the doctor. I doubt that it is the doctor.

The doctor wades through the list, talking to the "clients," writing a progress note and prescribing a pill and salutes "informed choice," during the fly by.

How many patients are on the list before the doctor is wearing the Emperor's New Clothes and merely posturing?

Reporting Bullying and Moral Injury?

Who is tasked with reporting bullying and moral injury in the healthcare workplace? The government has web sites, "stopbullying.gov," is an official government website designed to reduce bullying.

Osha addresses bullying in the workplace.
https://www.ccohs.ca/oshanswers/psychos
ocial/bullying.html

What is workplace bullying?

"Bullying is usually seen as acts or verbal comments that could psychologically or 'mentally' hurt or isolate a person in the workplace. Sometimes, bullying can involve negative physical contact as well. Bullying usually involves repeated incidents or a pattern of behavior that is intended to intimidate, offend, degrade, or humiliate a particular person or group of people. It has also been described as the assertion of power through aggression."

Health consequences of bullying in the healthcare workplace: A systematic review
医 护服务工作场所欺凌行为会带来的健康后果:系

统 性评价

Isabel Lever BA (Hons), MD, Daniel Dyball
BSc (Hons), Neil Greenberg MD, Sharon A.
M.
Stevelink PhD
First published: 28 February 2019
https://doi.org/10.1111/jan.13986Citations:
28

Theoretically anyone can, and everyone
should report bullying in the workplace.

It looks good on paper, but it really
doesn't work that way in the real world.

The Failure to Protect Whistleblowers?

"Frontline workers ...do not come forward
due to the fear of retaliation they have
and remain silent."

The Failures of Whistleblower Laws in
Protecting Workers - is unionization the
remedy to ensure compliance with cyber-
security laws? By Alvin Velazquez1 Sean
Hansen2 Despite all of these efforts,
frontline workers in the financial sector
and other sectors covered by the

patchwork of state and federal whistleblower laws do not come forward due to the fear of retaliation they have and remain silent.

"Whistleblowers are left open to retaliation despite new laws to protect them."

A FAILURE OF WHISTLEBLOWER PROTECTION

BROKEN GOVERNMENT

The Center for Public Integrity

Published — December 10, 2008Updated - May 19, 2014, at 12:19 pm ET

How America fails its whistleblowers who work with classified information have a few options. All of them are bad.

By Ranjani Chakraborty and Laura Bult

Nov 27, 2019, 10:00am EST

Why is it so difficult to provide informed choice in the medical setting?

Science has been corrupted by politics and money.

Pharmaceutical companies do not publish all the information necessary to provide informed choice.

Federal regulatory agencies have been captured by the pharmaceutical industry. Protecting Pharmaceutical Companies and the Revenue Streams of Pharmaceutical Companies has a priority over patient safety in federal regulatory agencies.

Protecting revenue streams in healthcare agencies has taken priority over patient safety.

Internal politics in healthcare agencies has taken priority over patient and staff safety.

Let me insert Old Wisdom here.

Old Wisdom has stood the test of time and has survived the rise and fall of empires, churches, fads, and hysterias for millennia.

First,
"No Good Deed Goes Unpunished."

Do not expect Whistleblower laws to protect you. Do not expect integrity from your chain of command. Be prepared to deal with antisocial personalities and antisocial behaviors in every setting that you find yourself in. Accept bullying as a condition of employment anywhere. Do not expect Good Deeds to be rewarded.

Second, Murphy's Law,

"Sooner or later if it can go wrong, it will go wrong."

If you see a risk in your workplace, know that it will happen sooner or later and you will be a part of the outcome, depending upon your behavior prior to the perfection of that risk in death or another bad outcome.

Do not expect any mercy from the plaintiff attorney.

Third, Pandora's Box.

Do not play with Pandora's Box.
Do not open Pandora's Box.
Once the evil in Pandora's box is released
it cannot be put back.

Just ask any president. The most
powerful person in the world cannot put
it back into Pandora's Box.

President Clinton famously said, "I did
not have sex with that woman."

President Nixon famously said, "I am not
a crook."

When attorneys get a hold of information
they will extract their pound of flesh,
Ford Motor company looked at Pinto
safety and The Pinto Memo: 'It's Cheaper
to let them Burn!' The result was
$128,000,000 in punitive damages
rendered by the jury.
https://www.spokesman.com/blogs/autos/2
008/o ct/17/pinto-memo-its-cheaper-let-
them-burn/

And

The Completely Preventable Disaster of
The Exploding Ford Pinto
T G Writes
Updated July 28, 2021
https://www.ranker.com/list/exploding-ford-pinto/tracey-graham

The Crisis in Science?

There has been a crisis in science for decades. Scientific research that is published can't be reproduced by other scientists.

Unless the research can be reproduced, it is not sound science.

1,500 scientists lift the lid on reproducibility Monya Baker nature news feature article Published: 25 May 2016
Nature volume 533, pages452–454 (2016)

The crisis in scientific publications is getting worse.

Interesting research is more likely to be published if it is interesting even if it is not science that can be replicated by other scientists.

"Papers that cannot be replicated are cited 153 times more because their findings are interesting, according to a new UC San Diego study."
A New Replication Crisis: Research that is Less Likely to be True is Cited More
May 21, 2021, | By Christine Clark
https://ucsdnews.ucsd.edu/pressrelease/a-new-replication-crisis-research-that-is-less-likely-be-true-is-cited-more?fbclid=IwAR3Eiqlm-hdMJTZ70FnhLv8WpMg5WrGTvnvX5aIlw x75dB4Qt OQon4jlnA

If a healthcare professional does not have the correct information, how is informed choice even possible?

Misinformation provided by
pharmaceutical companies.

It would seem that all businesses and
multinational corporations have a
tendency to promote bad science in
support of their revenue streams and
narratives.

The welfare of the public is a secondary
consideration for the purposes of window
dressing and deflection.

Trial sans Error: How Pharma-Funded
Research Cherry-Picks Positive Results
Clinical trial data on new drugs is
systematically withheld from doctors and
patients, bringing into question many of
the premises of the pharmaceutical
industry—and the medicine we use
By Ben Goldacre on February 13, 2013,
Published by Faber and Faber, Inc. © 2013
Ben Goldacre. Scientific American
https://www.scientificamerican.com/articl
e/trial -sans-error-how-pharma-funded-
research-cherry-picks-positive-results/

"The boundaries between academic medicine - medical schools, teaching hospitals, and their faculty - and the pharmaceutical industry have been dissolving since the 1980s, and the important differences between their missions are becoming blurred. Medical research, education, and clinical practice have suffered as a result."
Ex-editor of NEJM tells how Big Pharma has corrupted academic institutions
In the May/June issue of the Boston Review,
Dr. By Susan Perry

Federal Regulatory Agencies No Longer Protect American Citizens from Pharmaceutical Companies.

The FDA used to protect the United States Citizens from the Pharmaceutical industry.

An FDA director was decorated by President Kennedy for saving lives and protecting United States Citizens.

"President John F. Kennedy, in August 1962, awarding Dr. Frances Oldham Kelsey the President's Medal for Distinguished Federal Civilian Service for her exceptional judgment in evaluating the drug Thalidomide. Dr. Kelsey was only the second woman to receive this award—the highest honor that can be bestowed upon a US civilian"

Commemorative Issue: Protecting the Public:
Dr. Frances Oldham Kelsey
Karen Geraghty
AMA Journal of Ethics
Illuminating the Art of Medicine
Virtual Mentor. 2001;3(11):
DOI
10.1001 /virtualmentor.2001.3.11.prol2-0111.

A lot has changed since 1972.

50 years of approval? | FDA wants over half a century to disclose Pfizer jabs approval docs
https://www.youtube.com/watch?v=4u62p5KCFtE

FDA Says It Now Needs 75 Years to Fully Release Pfizer COVID-19 Vaccine Data Coronavirus, FDA, Pfizer, Coronavirus Vaccine Posted on All Sides December 8th, 2021 https://www.allsides.com/news/2021-12-08-1553 /fda-says-it-now-needs-75-years-fully-release-pfizer-covid-19-vaccine-data

Ivermectin is on the WHO (World Health Organization) list of safe and essential medications...ivermectin Tablet (scored): 3 mg https://apps.who.int/iris/bitstream/handle/1066 5/325771/WHO-MVP-EMP-IAU-2019.06-eng.pdf

"Conclusions:
Moderate-certainty evidence finds that large reductions in COVID-19 deaths are possible using ivermectin. Using ivermectin early in the clinical course may reduce numbers progressing to severe disease. The apparent safety and low cost suggest that ivermectin is likely to have a significant impact on the SARS-CoV-2 pandemic globally."

Ivermectin for Prevention and Treatment of COVID-19 Infection: A Systematic Review,

Meta-analysis, and Trial Sequential Analysis to Inform Clinical Guidelines

Bryant, Andrew MSc1, *; Lawrie, Theresa A. MBBCh, PhD2; Dowswell, Therese PhD; Fordham, Edmund J. PhD2; Mitchell, Scott MBChB, MRCS3; Hill, Sarah R. PhD1; Tham, Tony C. MD,

American Journal of Therapeutics: July/August 2021 - Volume 28 - Issue 4 - p e434-e460
THERAPEUTIC ADVANCES
doi: 10.1097/MJT.0000000000001402
https://journals.lww.com/americantherape utics/fulltext/2021/08000/ivermectin_for_pr evention_and_treatment_of.7.aspx

"Ivermectin fights 21 viruses, including SARS-CoV-2, the cause of Covid-19. A single dose reduced the viral load of SARS-CoV-2 in cells by 99.8% in 24 hours and 99.98% in 48 hours, according to a June 2020 study published in the journal Antiviral Research."

"In 115 patients with Covid-19 who received a single dose of ivermectin, none developed pneumonia or cardiovascular complications, while 11.4% of those in the control group did. Fewer ivermectin patients developed respiratory distress (2.6% vs. 15.8%); fewer required oxygen (9.6% vs. 45.9%); fewer required antibiotics (15.7% vs. 60.2%); and fewer entered intensive care (0.1% vs. 8.3%). Ivermectin-treated patients tested negative faster, in four days instead of 15, and stayed in the hospital nine days on average instead of 15. Ivermectin patients experienced 13.3% mortality compared with 24.5% in the control group."

"Despite the FDA's claims, ivermectin is safe at approved doses. Out of four billion doses administered since 1998, there have been only 28 cases of serious neurological adverse events, according to an article published this year in the American Journal of Therapeutics. The same study found that ivermectin has been used safely in pregnant women, children and infants."

Why Is the FDA Attacking a Safe,
Effective Drug?
Ivermectin is a promising Covid
treatment and prophylaxis, but the
agency is denigrating it. By David R.
Henderson and Charles L. Hooper July 28,
2021 12:34 pm ET
https://www.wsj.com/articles/fda-
ivermectin-cov id-19-coronavirus-masks-
anti-science-11627482 393

There is bad science, there is bullying in
health care, the pharmaceutical industry
promotes bad science, the federal
regulatory agencies protect the
pharmaceutical industry.

How does a clinician give informed
consent to a patient in real time?

In order to give the patient informed
consent, the physician must be able to tell
the patient what the risks and benefits of
the medication are.

The physician is often misinformed by the
medical literature for a variety of reasons.

First there is publication bias.
Publication bias
For a fact check and deeper look I refer
the reader to:
Publication bias in meta-analyses from
the Cochrane Database of Systematic
Reviews

Michal Kicinski David A. Springate
Evangelos
Kontopantelis

First published: 18 May 2015
https://doi.org/10.1002/sim.6525

For more information I refer the
reader to:
Not to be confused with Reporting bias or
Media bias. Publication bias is a type of
bias that occurs in published academic
research. It occurs when the outcome of
an experiment or research study
influences the decision whether to
publish or otherwise distribute it.
Publishing only results that show a
significant finding disturbs the balance of
findings and inserts bias in favor of
positive results.[1] The study of
publication bias is an important topic in

metascience. Studies with significant results can be of the same standard as studies with a null result with respect to quality of execution and design.[2] However, statistically significant results are three times more likely to be published than papers with null results.[3] A consequence of this is that researchers are unduly motivated to manipulate their practices to ensure that a statistically significant result is reported.[4]
From Wikipedia, the free encyclopedia.

I will leave it to the reader to research the following list of flaws in research regarding the risks and benefits of psychotropic medications.
Research fails to include pregnant women and children on ethical grounds.
Research fails to include elderly and people with multiple medical problems.
Research fails to include people on multiple medications.
Small sample size is not sufficient to provide reliable data.

Samples are not random because they do not include people who refuse.
Samples are not random because populations may not be accessible.
Studies are not randomized.
Studies are not blinded.
Studies do not use the same criteria for diagnosis or target symptoms.
The studies are of short duration.
Studies do not clearly separate spontaneous remission from medication effect.
Studies do not account for cognitive dissonance in addition to placebo effect.
It is difficult to identify altered data, "fudging."

This is not even the tip of the iceberg.

One study uncovered 710 unique research flaws for excluding research from evidence-based databases.

For fact checking and a deeper look at the shortcomings of medical research I refer the reader to:

A Large-Scale Analysis of the Reasons Given for Excluding Articles that are Retrieved by Literature Search During Systematic Review Tracy Edinger, ND, MCR and Aaron M. Cohen, MD, MS AMIA Annu Symp Proc. 2013; 2013: 379–387.
Published online 2013 Nov 16.
PMCID: PMC3900186
PMID: 24551345

Addicting Medications, No Functional Recovery The Long View
Your Nineteenth Psychiatric Consultation
William R. Yee M.D., J.D.
Copyright Applied for January 1st, 2021.

It is difficult for the physician to wade through an extensive medical literature and weed out the truth from the false research results being published.

"Considering that these surveys ask sensitive questions and have other limitations, it appears likely that this is a conservative estimate of the true prevalence of scientific misconduct."

How Many Scientists Fabricate and
Falsify Research? A Systematic Review
and Meta-Analysis of Survey Data
Daniele Fanelli
Published: May 29, 2009
https://doi.org/10.1371/journal.pone.000573
8

Prevalence of Research Misconduct and
Questionable Research Practices:
A Systematic Review and Meta-Analysis
Yu Xie, Kai Wang & Yan Kong
Practices: A Systematic Review and Meta-
Analysis. Sci Eng Ethics 27, 41 (2021).
https://doi.org/10.1007/s11948-021-00314-9
August 10, 2018 @@

"Findings
In this systematic review of 265 studies
comprising 400 647 drug samples and
meta-analysis of 96 studies comprising 67
839 drug samples, the prevalence of
substandard and falsified medicines in
low- and middle-income countries was
13.6% overall (19.1% for antimalarials and
12.4% for antibiotics). Data on the
estimated economic impact were limited

primarily to market size and ranged widely from $10 billion to $200 billion."

Prevalence and Estimated Economic Burden of Substandard and Falsified Medicines in Low- and Middle-Income Countries A Systematic
Review and Meta-analysis

Sachiko Ozawa, PhD, MHS,; Daniel R. Evans, MSc; Sophia Bessias, MPH; et al Deson G. Haynie, MHS; Tatenda T. Yemeke, MSc; Sarah K. Laing, MPH2; James E.
Herrington, PhD

JAMA Netw Open. 2018;1(4):e181662.
doi:10.1001/jamanetworkopen.2018.1662

"Both publication bias and outcome reporting bias may affect meta-analyses, and the effect can be unpredictable. Adding unreported data from both published and unpublished drug trials to 41 meta-analyses caused 46% of the meta-analytic effect estimates to show lower efficacy of the drug, 7% to show identical efficacy, and 46% to show greater efficacy." Preferred reporting items for

systematic review and meta-analysis protocols (PRISMA-P) 2015: elaboration and explanation
Larissa Shamseer, David Moher, Mike Clarke,
Davina Ghersi, Alessandro Liberati (deceased), Mark Petticrew, Paul Shekelle, Lesley A Stewart7the PRISMA-P Group
BMJ 2015; 349 doi:
https://doi.org/10.1136/bmj.g7647 (Published 02 January 2015)
Cite this as: BMJ 2015;349:g7647

Let us examine the antipsychotic medications.

An early large-scale examination of the effectiveness of antipsychotics was the CATIE trials.

Perphenazine is as effective as olanzapine, quetiapine, risperidone, and ziprasidone.

Perphenazine is the most cost-effective medication for the treatment of psychosis.

You can expect three out of four patients to stop antipsychotic medications within eighteen months due to side effects or failure of benefit to justify the time and money to continue the treatments. See:

"What CATIE Found: Results From the Schizophrenia Trial," Dr. Marvin S. Swartz, M.D., T. Scott Stroup, M.D., M.P.H., Dr. Joseph P. McEvoy, M.D., Dr. Sonia M. Davis, Dr.P.H., Dr. Robert A. Rosenheck, M.D., Dr. Richard S. E. Keefe, Ph.D., Dr. John K. Hsiao, M.D., and

Dr. Jeffrey A. Lieberman, M.D.; Psychiatr Serv.
2008 May; 59(5): 500–506.;
doi: 10.1176/ps.2008.59.5.500; PMCID: PMC5033643; NIHMSID: NIHMS816833; PMID: 18451005

There are many criticisms of the CATIE trials. See:
"CATIE & You, What happens when drugs are found to be unsafe and ineffective? Not much," by Ben Hansen,

The CATIE Schizophrenia Trial involved
1493 patients with schizophrenia treated
for up to 18 months with

olanzapine ....7.5 to 30 mg per day,
perphenazine ....8 to 32 mg per day,
quetiapine ....200 to 800 mg per day,
risperidone ....1.5 to 6.0 mg per day,
Ziprasidone ....40 to 160 mg per
day,

74 percent of patients discontinued
their medication before 18 months

64 percent of those assigned to olanzapine,
74 percent of those assigned to
perphenazine
82 percent of those assigned to quetiapine
74 percent of those assigned to
risperidone
79 percent of those assigned to
ziprasidone.

CONCLUSIONS

Patients discontinued medications for intolerable side effects or lack of benefit sufficient to justify the adverse effects and cost in time and money.

Effectiveness of Antipsychotic Drugs in Patients with Chronic Schizophrenia
Jeffrey A. Lieberman, M.D., T. Scott Stroup, M.D., M.P.H., Joseph P. McEvoy, M.D., Marvin S. Swartz, M.D., Robert A. Rosenheck, M.D., Diana O. Perkins, M.D., M.P.H., Richard S.E. Keefe, Ph.D., Sonia M. Davis, Dr.P.H., Clarence E. Davis, Ph.D., Barry D. Lebowitz,Ph.D., Joanne Severe, M.S., and John K. Hsiao, M.D.
September 22, 2005
N Engl J Med 2005; 353:1209-1223
DOI: 10.1056/NEJMoa051688

"Adverse effects are likely to be the most common reason for patients to not comply with prescribed medication regimens.

Ineffectiveness, complexity of the regimen and cost are also important medication-related factors contributing to noncompliance."

Noncompliance with Medication for Psychiatric Disorders
Reasons and Remedies
Robert Breen & Joshua T. Thornhill
Disease Management
Published: 14 September 2012
CNS Drugs volume 9, pages457–471 (1998)

"For example, the results of our recent telemedicine study, showed that the compliance rate, among schizophrenic patients with symptomatic remission, in the first month of the treatment was 44.6%, and had been decreasing over the subsequent 6 months (Krzystanek et al. 2015)."

RISK FACTORS FOR NONCOMPLIANCE WITH ANTIPSYCHOTIC MEDICATION IN LONG-TERM TREATED CHRONIC SCHIZOPHRENIA PATIENTS

Marek Krzystanek, Krzysztof Krysta, Maágorzata Janas-Kozik, Ewa Martyniak & Janusz Rybakowski

Psychiatria Danubina, 2019; Vol. 31, Suppl. 3, p 543-548 Conference paper ©

The standard of care is, "Informed Choice."

The best practice is, "the lowest effective dose."

Informed Choice requires that the psychiatrist inform the patient of the risks and benefits.

The lowest effective dose is the dose that gives the maximum benefit with the minimum side effect.

The Choice remains the patient's choice and not the doctor's choice.

The very concept of medication noncompliance is a violation of the standard of "Informed

Choice," as "Noncompliance," transfers the choice from the patient to the doctor.

If the patient finds the side effects unacceptable, then the lowest effective dose is no medication at all.

If the family, hospital, Peer Review, or other "stakeholder" is not satisfied with the patient's choice we are no longer in a doctor patient relationship.

The place of the "Stakeholders" in the equation needs to be evaluated through the lens of "Informed Choice," and "the lowest effective dose."

Which stakeholder has the power to impose his or her will on the patient?

Is it the spouse, parent, child, teacher, Peer Review Committee, State Licensing Board, Credentialling Committee, Malpractice Insurance Carrier?

I will let each reader decide for themselves.

Corporate America has a long history of lying, cheating and stealing to boost profits.

I refer the reader to the following:

In the best of all possible worlds, science should provide a guide for progress of political, business, and social evolution.

However, in the real world, politics and business corrupt science and political evolution.

The sugar industry actively redirected science, politics and social evolution away from the risks of sugar, obesity, diabetes and heart disease to red meat and fat.

For a fact check and a deeper look I refer the reader to
50 Years Ago, Sugar Industry Quietly Paid Scientists To Point Blame At Fat
September 13, 20169:59 AM ET
CAMILA DOMONOSKE
and:

Sugar Industry and Coronary Heart
Disease Research
A Historical Analysis of Internal
Industry Documents

Cristin E. Kearns, DDS, MBA1,2; Laura A.
Schmidt, PhD, MSW, MPH1,3,4; Stanton A.
Glantz, PhD1,5,6,7,8
Author Affiliations

JAMA Intern Med. 2016;176(11):1680-1685.
doi:10.1001/jamainternmed.2016.5394
November 2016

This was not a first, but a part of a long
history of big business creating fake
science to support a revenue stream.

For a fact check and deeper look I refer
the reader to the asbestos coverup:
Review:
The Dusting of America: A Story of
Asbestos: Carnage, Cover-Up, and
Litigation
Reviewed Work: Outrageous Misconduct:
The Asbestos Industry on Trial
by Paul Brodeur
Review by: David Rosenberg
Harvard Law Review

Vol. 99, No. 7 (May, 1986), pp. 1693-1706 (14 pages)
Published By: The Harvard Law Review Association
https://doi.org/10.2307/1341085
https://www.jstor.org/stable/1341085

For a fact check and deeper look into the Tobacco Industry I refer the reader to:
Smokescreen: The Truth Behind the Tobacco Industry Cover-up
Robert N. Proctor, PhD
Author Affiliations
JAMA. 1996;276(12):998.
doi:10.1001/jama.1996.03540120076040
September 25, 1996

The pharmaceutical industry has a long record of misinformation and abuse of the market place.

For a fact check and deeper look into Neurontin/gabapentin I refer the reader to:
Pfizer to Pay $420 Million in Illegal Marketing Case
By Kenneth N. Gilpin

New York Times
May 13, 2004

In regards a fact check and deeper look
into illegal marketing and pleading guilty
to criminal charges I refer the reader to:
"In May 2004, Pfizer agreed to pay $430
million and to plead guilty to criminal
charges for illegally marketing Neurontin
for unapproved uses such as migraine
headaches and pain."
Pfizer to pay $325 million in Neurontin
settlement
By Jonathan Stempe JUNE 2, 20149:55 AM
UPDATED 7 YEARS AGO
For a fact check and deeper look into
Oxycontin I refer the reader to:
OxyContin maker Purdue Pharma pleads
guilty to criminal charges
HEALTHCARE & PHARMA
NOVEMBER 24, 2020; 12:10 PMU PDATED
12
DAYS AGO
By Mike Spector
 and:

OxyContin Maker To Pay Out Billions In
Civil, Criminal Penalties
October 22, 2020 5:06 AM ET
LAW NPR
Heard on Morning Edition
BRIAN MAN
Addicting Medications, No Functional
Recovery, The Long View Your
Nineteenth Psychiatric Consultation
William R. Yee M.D., J.D.
Copyright Applied for January 1st, 2021

In my office it is
"Informed Choice," and,
"The Lowest Effective Dose," and the
arbiter of those issues is:
the client and:
the client only.

Let us examine the process
of informed choice.

The client is examined and diagnosed
with schizophrenia, schizoaffective
disorder, bipolar disorder, depression
with psychotic symptoms, or a diagnosis
with hallucinations, delusions and or

paranoia appropriate for antipsychotic medications.

The diagnosis cannot be confirmed by x-ray, blood test, or other basis that is as specific as the identification of a bacteria in pneumonia.

The diagnosis is a guess based upon a collection of symptoms, but the cause is not known.

Because we really don't know what mental illness is on the same sound basis that we know what bacterial pneumonia is, we cannot know what the mechanism of action of antipsychotic medication is. "The dopamine hypothesis of schizophrenia postulates that postsynaptic dopamine antagonism is the common mechanism that explains antipsychotic properties."

The dopamine hypothesis of schizophrenia embraces the thought that first-generation (typical) antipsychotics are D2 antagonists.

The dopamine hypothesis of schizophrenia embraces the thought that second-generation antipsychotics include 5-HT2A antagonism, fast D2 dissociation, and 5-HT1A agonism.

Mechanism of Action of Antipsychotic Agents

Flavio Guzman, M.D.

Psychopharmacology Institute
https://psychopharmacologyinstitute.com/publication/mechanism-of-action-of-antipsychotic-agents-2094

"The mechanism of action of most first- and second-generation antipsychotics (FGAs and SGAs) appears to be postsynaptic blockade of brain dopamine D2 receptors."

Second-generation antipsychotic medications: Pharmacology, administration, and side effects

Author: Michael D Jibson, MD, PhD. Section

Editor: Stephen Marder, MD Deputy Editor: Michael Friedman, MD

You offer the client a choice of
medications and advise the patient that:
Discontinuation rates for antipsychotics
are
.....olanzapine 64%
.....risperidone ...74%
.....perphenazine 75%
.....ziprasidone ...79%

From the patient's perspective
the psychiatrist must treat
3 patients with olanzapine
for 1 patient to get better
4 patients with risperidone
for 1 patient to get better
4 patients with perphenazine
for 1 patient to get better
5 patients with ziprasidone
for 1 patient to get better
sufficiently for the patient to be willing
to continue the medication.

The CATIE Schizophrenia Trial: Results,
Impact, Controversy
Theo C. Manschreck , MD, MPH &Roger A.
Boshes , MD, PhD
Pages 245-258 | Received 16 Mar 2007,
Accepted 15 Jun 2007, Published online:

03 Jul 2009

Then you introduce the patient to the concept of NNH, the Number Needed to Harm.

Doctors lack information about how often patients suffer side effects. For this reason doctors lack the ability to give complete information for informed choice.

Doctors cannot tell patients how many patients are treated with a medication for one patient to suffer harm. NNH is the number of patients treated for one patient to suffer harm.

It has been known for decades that medication side effects, including death, are underreported.
For 60 years, underreporting has plagued the FDA system for tracking drug side effects
John Fauber, Milwaukee Journal Sentinel
https://www.jsonline.com/story/news/inves
tigations/2020/11/30/underreporting-has-

Haloperidol therapy with dementia may be associated with 1 additional death for every 26 patients receiving treatment.

NNH is 26 with death being the harm.

Haloperidol had the highest risk of death and quetiapine had the least risk of death.

Risperidone and olanzapine increased the death rate more than quetiapine.

Finally higher doses of antipsychotics have higher death rates.

Quetiapine increased mortality by 2.0%, yielding an NNH of 50

Quetiapine has the least mortality, but less benefit than olanzapine or risperidone.
Antipsychotics, Other Psychotropics, and the Risk of Death in Patients With Dementia Number Needed to Harm

Donovan T. Maust, MD, MS; Hyungjin
Myra
Kim, ScD; Lisa S. Seyfried, MD, MS; et al
Claire Chiang, PhD; Janet Kavanagh, MS;
Lon
S. Schneider, MD, MS; Helen C. Kales,
MD Author Affiliations Article
Information
JAMA Psychiatry.
2015;72(5):438-445.
doi:10.1001/jamapsychiatry.2014.3018

There is a Block Box Warning in the FDA
labels for antipsychotic medications
because it is known that antipsychotics
cause death in elderly patients with
dementia.

What about the elderly without dementia?

Are antipsychotic medications safe with
the elderly without dementia?

"Conclusions
Prevalence of potentially inappropriate
medications in nursing homes according
to the NORGEP-NH was extensive, and
especially the use of multiple

psychotropic drugs. The high prevalence found in this study shows that there is a need for higher awareness of medication use and side effects in the elderly population."

Potentially inappropriate medication use in nursing homes: an observational study using the NORGEP-NH criteria

Gunhild Nyborg, Mette Brekke, Jørund Straand, Svein Gjelstad, and Maria Romøren BMC Geriatr. 2017; 17: 220. Published online 2017 Sep 19. doi: 10.1186/s12877-017-0608-z PMCID: PMC5606129 PMID: 28927372

"Conclusions
This study found that psychiatric patients in contact with a CMHS have an almost twofold higher mortality rate than the general population. These findings demonstrate that, since the closure of long-stay psychiatric hospitals, the physical health care of people with mental health problems is often neglected and clearly requires greater attention by

health-care policymakers, services and professionals."
Mortality and cause of death among psychiatric patients: a 20-year case-register study in an area with a community-based system of care
L. Grigoletti, G. Perini, A. Rossi, A. Biggeri, C. Barbui, M. Tansella and F. Amaddeo
Published online by Cambridge University Press: 20 April 2009

"The FDA black box warning that use of atypical antipsychotic medications in elderly patients with dementia nearly doubled the risk of death, clinicians, patients and caregivers are left with unclear choices for treating people with dementia with psychosis and/or severe agitation."
Antipsychotic treatments for the elderly: efficacy and safety of aripiprazole
Izchak Kohen, Paula E Lester, and Sum Lam Neuropsychiatr Dis Treat. 2010; 6: 47–58.
Published online 2010 Mar 24. doi: 10.2147/ndt.s6411
PMCID: PMC2846120

PMID: 20361061

Elderly patients with schizophrenia are a particularly vulnerable group often excluded from clinical trials.
Currently there is no evidence-synthesis about the efficacy and safety of antipsychotics in this subgroup."
Antipsychotic drugs for elderly patients with schizophrenia: A systematic review and meta-analysis

Marc Krause 1, Maximilian Huhn , Johannes
Schneider-Thoma , Philipp Rothe , Robert C Smith 3, Stefan Leucht
Affiliations expand

Meta-Analysis Eur Neuropsychopharmacol.
2018 Dec;28(12):1360-1370. doi: 10.1016/j.euroneuro.2018.09.007. Epub 2018 Sep 20.
PMID: 30243680 DOI: 10.1016/j.euroneuro.2018.09.007

"There is no trial-based evidence upon which to base guidelines for the treatment of late-onset schizophrenia."

Antipsychotic drug treatment for elderly
people with late-onset schizophrenia
Adib Essali 1, Ghassan Ali
Review Cochrane Database Syst Rev.
2012 Feb 15; 2012(2):CD004162.
doi:10.1002/14651858.CD004162.pub2.
PMID: 22336800 PMCID: PMC6986693
DOI: 10.1002/14651858.CD004162.pub2

The bottom line is that there is no basis
for concluding that antipsychotic
medication is safer to use in the elderly
without dementia than elderly patients
with dementia.

The elderly, in general, have declining
physiologic reserves and tolerate adverse
medication effects less than the young
and healthy. That is why the elderly are
more likely to die with the flu or a
pandemic.

**Another measure of the benefit is what
percentage of symptoms are removed in
response to the medication. The range is
zero percent, 0%, to one hundred percent,**

100%. Zero would be no benefit and one hundred percent would be a cure.
For psychotropic medications 20% reduction of symptoms is sufficient for the FDA to give approval for marketing the medication for the treatment of mental illness.

A 40% reduction of symptoms is a "robust," response from the point of view of the pharmaceutical industry.

The pharmaceutical industry is interested in a revenue stream and there is a great temptation to lie, steal and cheat based upon the fines and criminal prosecutions listed above.

From the viewpoint of the patient, family and significant others a cure is desired.

Twenty to forty percent reduction of symptoms is not a cure and fifty to seventy five percent of patients stop taking psychotropic medications after eighteen months.

Is that fifty to seventy five percent who stop taking antipsychotic medications properly classified as noncompliance or a vote of no confidence.

Clozaril-Clozapine

Let us examine Clozaril, a putative "Gold Standard," in the treatment of severe mental illness, especially Schizophrenia.

Clozaril is prescribed when mentally ill patients fail to respond to other antipsychotic medications.

Let us examine some of the available literature on Clozaril.

Keep in mind there is a replication crisis in science, there is publication bias, bad research is more likely to be cited and found than good research, pharmaceutical companies often publish misleading research or present and most importantly, side effects are under reported as cited above.

Results

A total of 108 studies revealed an incidence of clozapine-associated

neutropenia..3.8%
severe neutropenia..................................0.9%
Death was..0.013%
Fatality of severe neutropenia was..2.1%

The prevalence of agranulocytosis and related death in clozapine-treated patients: a comprehensive meta-analysis of observational studies

Published online by Cambridge University
Press: 12 March 2019

Xiao-Hong Li,, Xiao-Mei Zhong,, Li Lu, Wei Zheng,, Shi-bin Wang,, Wen-wang Rao

Background

Clozapine treatment increases the risk of agranulocytosis, but the epidemiology of agranulocytosis has been inconsistent.

Results

Studies with 260,948 clozapine-treated patients published between 1984 and 2018 reveal:

prevalence of agranulocytosis 0.4%
death caused by agranulocytosis... ..0.05%

The prevalence of agranulocytosis and related death in clozapine-treated patients: a comprehensive meta-analysis of observational studies

Xiao-Hong Li, Xiao-Mei Zhong, Li Lu, Wei Zheng, Shi-Bin Wang, Wen-Wang Rao, Shuai Wang, Chee H Ng, Gabor S Ungvari, Gang Wang, Yu-Tao Xiang

Meta-Analysis Psychol Med. 2020 Mar;50(4):583-594. doi: 10.1017/S0033291719000369.
Epub 2019 Mar 12.
PMID: 30857568 DOI: 10.1017/S0033291719000369

Clozapine treated patients who suffered sudden death were about 10 years younger and healthier than non Clozapine treated patients who experienced sudden death.

The sudden death rate was 3.8 times higher for Clozapine treated patients than for nonclozapine treated patients, whereas the rate of disease-related death was 5 times higher for nonclozapine treated patients than for clozapine treated patients.

The rate of suicide among patients currently receiving clozapine in this sample was 3.6 times higher than among nonclozapine treated patients.

Because clozapine treated patients who experienced sudden death were also younger and healthier, it seems that treatment with clozapine may present a greater risk for sudden death than treatment with other psychiatric medications.

Sudden death in patients receiving clozapine treatment: a preliminary investigation

I Modai, S Hirschmann, A Rava, R Kurs, P Barak, P Lichtenberg, M Ritsner Case Reports J Clin Psychopharmacol. 2000 Jun;20(3):325-7.
PMID: 10831019
DOI: 10.1097/00004714-200006000-00006

Mortality rate ratios were not significantly lower in patients ever treated with clozapine during follow-up, but significantly lower in patients continuously treated with clozapine compared to patients with other antipsychotics Potentially fatal outcomes associated with clozapine

Kevin J. Liabc, Ronald J. Gurreraabc, Lynn
E. Delisiabc

Schizophrenia Research
Volume 199, September 2018, Pages 386-389

Abstract
Morbidity and mortality associated with clozapine includes risk of agranulocytosis, aspiration pneumonia, bowel ischemia, myocarditis, seizures, and weight gain. Mortality with clozapine induced myocarditis can be 24%.
Long term all-cause mortality can be 22%. About 43% were diagnosed with diabetes compared to a national prevalence of 13.7%. Clozapine can cause death by

cardiovascular and other medical disorders.

Clozapine, Diabetes Mellitus, Cardiovascular Risk and Mortality: Results of a 21-Year Naturalistic Study in Patients with Schizophrenia and Schizoaffective Disorder

Katlyn L Nemani, M Claire Greene, Melissa Ulloa, Brenda Vincenzi, Paul M Copeland, Sulaiman Al-Khadari, David C Henderson

PMID: 29164928 PMCID: PMC6489443 DOI: 10.3371/CSRP.KNMG.111717

There is not a scientific basis to determine which antipsychotic is more effective for patients with treatment-resistant schizophrenia. Blinded Random Controlled Trials in contrast to unblinded, randomized effectiveness studies do not provide evidence of the superiority of clozapine compared with other second-generation antipsychotics"

Efficacy, Acceptability, and Tolerability of Antipsychotics in Treatment-Resistant Schizophrenia: A Network Meta-analysis

Myrto T Samara, Markus Dold, Myrsini

ianatsi, Adriani Nikolakopoulou, Bartosz Helfer, Georgia Salanti, Stefan Leucht Meta-Analysis JAMA Psychiatry. 2016 Mar;73(3):199-210. doi: 10.1001/jamapsychiatry.2015.2955. PMID: 26842482 DOI: 10.1001/jamapsychiatry.2015.2955

Clinicians must monitor WBC and granulocyte counts and may wish to consider weekly hematologic monitoring for the duration of clozapine therapy. Abrupt agranulocytosis may occur at any time.

Sudden Late Onset of Clozapine-Induced Agranulocytosis

Nick C Patel, Peter G Dorson, Tawny L Bettinger
First Published June 1, 2002 Case Report
Find in PubMed
https://doi.org/10.1345/aph.1A417

"There are two major classes of ADRs (ADR is Adverse Drug Reaction) : (1) unpredictable, uncommon and idiosyncratic, and (2) predictable, common and dose-related [4]. The latter

are better described as related to serum concentrations [5]. There is recent agreement among the most important medical scientists, such as Vanderbroucke and Psaty [6] or Ioannidis [7], that the status of ADR science is highly deficient._ According to them, there are two main reasons for the poor status of ADR knowledge [6, 7]: (1) pharmaceutical companies tend to try to minimize the existence of ADRs, and (2) rare but potentially lethal ADRs, usually idiosyncratic, are usually not detected by the randomized clinical trials (RCTs) required for drug approval, since they are short-term and include only a few thousand patients. These deficiencies have led to several drugs being withdrawn from the market due to unidentified potentially lethal ADRs [8]."
A Rational Use of Clozapine Based on Adverse Drug Reactions, Pharmacokinetics, and Clinical Pharmacopsychology
de Leon J., Ruan C.J.d, Schoretsanitis G., De las Cuevas C.

Psychother Psychosom 2020;89:200–214
https://doi.org/10.1159/000507638

Clozapine-Clozaril through the lens of the FDA Label

The FDA Label is the most convenient and comprehensive source of information available to the practicing clinician for the evaluation and use of medications. That FDA Label for most medications will list hundreds of effects and side effects including:
Black Box warnings for death in demented geriatric paitients.
Birth Defects
Myocarditis
Leukopenia
Neuroleptic Malignant Syndrome
Constipation
Tardive Dyskinisia
Toxic Symptoms of Overdose
Withdrawal Syndromes-Rebound Symptoms Literally hundreds of side effects

Let us examine the FDA Label for Clozaril as a tool for giving the patient informed choice.

This is done knowing that side effects are under reported and pharmaceutical companies have a history of exaggerating benefits and minimizing side effects in research data.

I leave it to the reader to determine how much the benefits are exaggerated and how much the adverse effects are minimized.

I have not found the perfect method for sorting these matters out, after fifty years as a practicing physician, with diligence in monitoring the literature and educating patients about medications.

I start by telling the patient that they should report all new physical symptoms as any symptom can be a medication side effect, previously known, or waiting to be discovered

Second, I tell my patients that with psychiatric medications, the safest thing to do if a side effect emerges is to stop the medications, go to an emergency room for serious side effects and or make an appointment to adjust medications for minor side effects.

The client is stuck with determining what a serious, life-threatening side effect is.

I suggest rash, itching, difficulty breathing, difficulty maintaining consciousness and rational thinking are likely to be emergencies.

I suggest that the client read the package insert for a list of side effects or look the for FDA label online. If the client is in my office, I will give the client a copy of the FDA Label and review it with them.
The FDA Label for Clozaril reports:
BOXED WARNING
1. AGRANULOCYTOSIS
2. SEIZURES
3. MYOCARDITIS
4. OTHER ADVERSE CARDIOVASCULAR

AND RESPIRATORY EFFECTS
5. INCREASED MORTALITY IN ELDERLY
PATIENTS WITH DEMENTIA-
RELATED PSYCHOSIS

I will advise the patient that there is no sound basis for believing that Clozaril/Clozapine is safer in elderly patients without dementia.

I will advise the patient that physiologic reserves decline with age and with chronic medical conditions such as obesity, diabetes, high blood pressure and other medical abnormalities.

Additional Risks include:
1. Hyperglycemia and Diabetes Mellitus
2. Neuroleptic Malignant Syndrome (NMS)
3. Neuroleptic Malignant Syndrome (NMS)
4. Fever
5. Pulmonary Embolism
6. Hepatitis
7. Anticholinergic Toxicity
8. fecal impaction and paralytic

9. anticholinergic effects aggravating
    prostatic enlargement
10. Interference with Cognitive and Motor
 Performance
11. Cerebrovascular adverse events

Pregnancy Category B
The effects on pregnancy are not
adequately studied and unknown and the
medication should be avoided as much as
possible during pregnancy.

OVERDOSAGE
Human Experience The most commonly
reported signs and symptoms associated
with CLOZARIL® (clozapine) overdose
are: altered states of consciousness,
including drowsiness, delirium and coma;
tachycardia; hypotension; respiratory
depression or failure; hypersalivation.
Aspiration pneumonia and cardiac
arrhythmias have also been reported.
Seizures have occurred in a minority of
reported cases.
Fatal overdoses have been reported with
CLOZARIL, at doses above 2500 mg. There
have also been reports of patients

recovering from overdoses well in excess of 4 g.

After the client is educated as to the risks of Clozapine, the client is educated as to benefits of Clozapine.

According to the Clozapine FDA Label The effectiveness of CLOZARIL in a treatment-resistant schizophrenic population was demonstrated in a 6-week study comparing CLOZARIL and chlorpromazine.

Patients meeting DSM-III criteria for schizophrenia and having a mean BPRS total score of 61 were demonstrated to be treatment resistant by history and by open, prospective treatment with haloperidol before entering into the double-blind phase of the study.

The superiority of CLOZARIL to chlorpromazine was documented in statistical analyses employing both categorical and continuous measures of treatment effect "Patients who met the multiple psychiatric symptom criteria were then randomly assigned to a six-week double-blind treatment trial with either clozapine (up to 900 mg/d) or chlorpromazine and benztropine mesylate (up to 1800 mg/d of chlorpromazine hydrochloride and up to 6 mg of Benztropine mesylate)."

"Average daily doses of active antipsychotic medication received during double-blind treatment are shown by treatment week in Fig 1. Adequate dose levels of each drug were attained with mean peak dosages exceeding 1200 mg/d of chlorpromazine and 600 mg/d of clozapine. The decrease in average dosage for both treatment groups at week 6 reflects the mandated taper-down at the end of the treatment period for all patients, designed to avoid abrupt discontinuation."

BPRS total score C
Clozapine ....126 Patients
Baseline Score   61 ±12
Endpoint Score 45 ± 13
Chlorpromazine ....139 Patients
Baseline Score   61 ±11
Endpoint Score   56 ± 12
Two-Tailed Analysis of Covariance, P
< .001

BPRS cluster of four key items
Clozapine ....126 Patients
Baseline Score 19 ± 04
Endpoint Score 14 ± 05
Chlorpromazine 139 Patients
Baseline Score 19 ± 04
Endpoint Score 17 ± 04
 Two-Tailed Analysis of Covariance, P
< .001

The criteria for defining a patient as
improved reduction greater than 20%
from baseline in the BPRS total score
plus
a posttreatment CGI Scale score of
3 (mild) or less
or

a posttreatment BPRS total score of
35 or lower

It was found that only
4% of patients treated with
chlorpromazine and benztropine had
improved, while
30% of clozapine-treated patients had
improved.
Clozapine for the treatment-resistant
schizophrenic. A double-blind comparison
with chlorpromazine
J Kane 1, G Honigfeld, J Singer, H Meltzer
Clinical Trial Arch Gen Psychiatry 1988
Sep;45(9):789-96. doi:
10.1001/archpsyc.1988.01800330013001.
PMID: 3046553 DOI:
10.1001/archpsyc.1988.01800330013001

My first comment is that there is a
large subjective element involved in
the BPRS. A total of 265 severely
mentally ill patients were found with
an average baseline score of 61 with a
plus minus of 11 or 12.

A total of 265 patients were found with a score of 19 plus minus 4 on four key indicators.

First you must know what a BPRS Score is.

BPRS is short for Brief Psychiatric Rating Scale

The rater is asked to render his opinion on 18 aspects of mental illness.

From a range of zero to seven, least to worst he will give his opinion on the severity of each aspect of mental illness in the BPRS That means the range of scores is from 0 to 126.

My second comment is that based upon this I should inform my patients that if they want to accept a therapeutic trial of Clozapine, they can expect a 30% chance of a 20% improvement.

The client can expect 3 out of ten patients to benefit from clozapine. That is about 1

out of 3 patients will benefit by taking
Clozaril.

I suppose if the client thought the mental
illness was very severe, the client might
be willing to accept death as an
alternative to mental illness.

The adverse effects of Clozaril include
severe physical illness and death. The risk
is so high that the patient must accept
weekly blood tests to continue taking the
Clozaril.

Because of the severity of adverse effects,
treatment of patients failing to show a
clinically significant response should not
continue

What is a clinically significant response?

Ask the patient.

The need for continuing treatment in
patients with clinical responses should be
periodically reevaluated.

The client should be offered a medication taper as an option with each visit to determine the continued need for clozapine. It is always the patient's choice based upon the patient's willingness to accept risks for benefits.

Thank you for your time and attention.
William R. Yee M.D., J.D.
Board Certified Psychiatrist.
Practicing Medicine and Psychiatry without interruption since 1972 in Michigan, Indiana, Kentucky, California and Texas

"Pre-Existing text," includes names of Symptoms and medical illnesses, medications, people, corporations, law cases, statutes, text of statutes, the titles of articles and books, the content of articles and books cited.

My copyright claim is a clam to the
"original text," which is my personal
experiences as described in the text
above and my commentary on the names
of symptoms and medical illnesses,
medications, people, corporations, law
cases, statutes, text of statutes, the titles
of articles and books, the content of
articles and books cited.